Dash Diet Cookbook

A Complete Dash Diet Program With 30 Days Meal Plan And 50+ Healthy Recipes For Weight Loss And Lowering Blood Pressure

D1441581

© **Copyright 2019 by**_____

All rights reserved.

The following eBook is reproduced below with the goal of providing information that is as accurate and reliable as possible. Regardless, purchasing this e-book can be seen as consent to the fact that both the publisher and the author of this book are in no way experts on the topics discussed within and that any recommendations or suggestions that are made herein are for entertainment purposes only. Professionals should be consulted as needed prior to undertaking any of the action endorsed herein.

This declaration is deemed fair and valid by both the American Bar Association and the Committee of Publishers Association and is legally binding throughout the United States.

Furthermore, the transmission, duplication, or reproduction of any of the following work including specific information will be considered an illegal act irrespective of if it is done electronically or in print. This extends to creating a secondary or tertiary copy of the work or a recorded copy and is only allowed with an express written consent from the Publisher. All additional rights reserved.

The information in the following pages is broadly considered a truthful and accurate account of facts. As such, any inattention, use, or misuse of the information in question by the reader will render any resulting actions solely under their purview. There are no scenarios in which the publisher or the original author of this work can be in any fashion deemed liable for any hardship or damages that may befall them after undertaking information described herein.

Additionally, the information in the following pages is intended only for informational purposes and should thus be thought of as universal. As befitting its nature, it is presented without assurance regarding its prolonged validity or interim quality. Trademarks that are mentioned are done without written consent and can in no way be considered an endorsement from the trademark holder.

CONTETNS

INTRODUCTION

DASH diet or Dietary Approaches to Stop Hypertension is a lifetime method to healthy eating. This diet program is intended to prevent hypertension whilst encourage one to take on the low sodium diet.

What to eat?

Here's a rundown of the suggested serving sizes for a 2,000 calorie DASH diet.

Grains – this includes bread, pasta, and rice. Whole grains are recommended because they contain more nutrients and fiber weigh against the refined version. For instance, eat brown rice, whole-wheat pasta, and whole-grain bread instead of white rice, regular pasta, and white bread. When shopping for food, always look for 100% whole wheat and whole grain.

In a day, you're allowed to eat grains of at least one serving, ½ cup cereal (cooked), one slice of whole wheat bread, ½ cup pasta, or ½ cup rice.

Fruits – you are allowed to consume at least 4 servings in a day. You may portion your fruit consumption by snacking ½ cup of fresh fruits in the morning, a serving of 1 medium-sized fruit in the afternoon, and 4 ounces any fruit juice of choice as an afternoon snack, and another ½ cup of canned or frozen fruit in the evening. For fruit juices, make sure that you go for freshly squeezed ones. If you're buying canned fruits, ensure that there is no sugar added.

Vegetables – 4 servings are allowed in the Dash diet. Example servings include 1 cup of cooked or raw vegetables. Both frozen and fresh vegetables are excellent vegetable sources. However, when you buy canned or frozen veggies, make sure that they are low in sodium. In order to increase the number of servings of vegetables in a day, you have to be creative in your cooking. In the morning, you may have stir-fried mixed vegetables, during lunch time, you can have steamed vegetables, fresh carrots and celery sticks during snack time, and vegetables with a slice of chicken breast for dinner. Just remember to double up the amount of veggies instead of meat.

Protein – you can go for poultry, lean meat, and fish. It is advised that you consume at least 4-6 servings of any of these. Opt for the leaner versions and servings should be no more than 6 oz in a day. For cooking, grilling, baking, and broiling instead of frying are suggested.

Dairy – you can have at least 2 servings of this in a day. If you're going to have milk, cheese, or yogurt, ensure that they are fat free or low in fat. Example serving is 1 cup skim milk, 1 1/2 oz cheese (part-skim) or 1 cup yogurt (low fat).

Whether you're already doing the DASH diet or you're still planning to do it, here are some tips on how to get started and stay on track:

⌂⃗✍ List everything before you head to the supermarket

If you want to be consistent in your diet, everything should begin with your food. So before you go to the grocery, it is important that you:

- ✓ Create a checklist - this includes all the meals and ingredients that you're going to make for the coming days or for a whole week. It would also be easier to indicate if the meal is for breakfast, lunch, dinner, or snacks. With all these listed, it's less likely that you'll grab unhealthy food.

- ✓ Make sure your stomach is full before heading to the grocery – this is because when you go there hungry, all food that you see will look appealing to you especially those high in sodium nd fat.

📄✍ Always keep the DASH diet in mind

When going grocery shopping, it is but normal to be tempted to go to bargain sales, but just as you would want to get a discount on these, most food on this rack are prohibited in the Dash diet as they are mostly sugary and have too much salt.

⊟☞   Always go for the fresh ones

Most food that are high in sodium are the processed ones. Fresh food are definitely healthier options because only a little sugar, fat, and sodium are added. Fresh food also contain natural vitamins and minerals weigh against the frozen, canned, and processed ones.

⊟☞   Make it a habit to read the labels all the time

The Nutrition facts at the back of each food item is there for good reason. When reading labels, look for reduced fat and sodium products. Choose the ones lower in fat and sodium, and those with fewer calories.

⊟☞   Shop the sides

Fresh produce, lean meats, and low-fat products are always found at the sides. Those at the center aisles are mostly prohibited in the dash diet.

30-DAY MEAL PLAN

Day 1

Breakfast - French Toast

Lunch - Baked Marinara Turkey Meatball

Dinner – Gourmet Potato and Asparagus Salad

Desserts/ Snacks - Nutty Banana Muffins

Day 2

Breakfast – Whole Wheat Hotcakes

Lunch – Asparagus and Prosciutto in Vinegar

Dinner – Spareribs with Ginger Sauce

Desserts/Snacks - Broccoli and Turkey Muffin

Day 3

Breakfast – Cheesy Egg and Spinach on Wheat Toast

Lunch – Roasted Asparagus with Herbs and Feta Cheese

Dinner – Roasted Mint Tomato Soup

Desserts/Snacks - Baked Sweet Potato Crisps

Day 4

Breakfast – Nutty Banana Pancakes

Lunch – Angel Kale Puttanesca

Dinner – Burrito Salad in a Jar

Desserts/Snacks - Baked Sweet Potato Crisps

Day 5

Breakfast – Nutty Banana Pancakes

Lunch – Angel Kale Puttanesca

Dinner – Zucchini, Spinach, and Tomatoes Soup

Desserts/Snacks – Banana, Apple, and Chia Seed Parfait

Day 6

Breakfast – Whole Wheat Pasta and Chicken

Lunch – Creamy Tomato Broccoli

Dinner – Pumpkin Soup with Macadamia Cheese

Desserts/Snacks – Avocado Quesadillas

Day 7

Breakfast – Scramble Tofu with Herbs

Lunch – Sweet Potato Salad in Balsamic Vinegar

Dinner – Sweet Potato and Roasted Pepper Soup

Desserts/Snacks - Pumpkin Biscuits

Day 8

Breakfast – Blueberry Oatmeal

Lunch – Curried Chicken

Dinner – Penne Pasta with Kale

Desserts/Snacks - Granola

Day 9

Breakfast – Mixed Green Fruits Juice

Lunch – Grilled Cauliflower

Dinner – Arugula, Corn Kernels Salad

Desserts/Snacks – Blueberry Muffins

Day 10

Breakfast – Broccoli Omelet

Lunch – Heirloom Tomatoes and Ruby Beets Salad

Dinner – Apple Pork Stew

Desserts/Snacks – Egg Rolls with Lime Avocado Dip

Day 11

Breakfast – Spanish-Inspired Scrambled Egg

Lunch – Kale and Mango Salad

Dinner – Apple Pork Stew

Desserts/Snacks – Pumpkin Pie

Day 12

Breakfast – Peaches Kiwi Shake

Lunch – Wheat Tortillas with Peppers and Mushrooms

Dinner – Mexican-Style Salad

Desserts/Snacks – All Fruits Salad

Day 13

Breakfast – Cashew Date and Coconut Smoothie

Lunch – Wheat Tortillas with Peppers and Mushrooms

Dinner – Radish, Baby Greens, and Cucumber Salad -

Desserts/Snacks – All Fruits Salad

Day 14

Breakfast – Lettuce, Avocado, and Chicken Salad

Lunch – Wheat Tortillas with Peppers and Mushrooms

Dinner – Watercress, Fennel, and Apple Salad

Desserts/Snacks – Avocado with Ginger Smoothie

Day 15

Breakfast – French Toast

Lunch – Baked Marinara Turkey Meatball

Dinner – Gourmet Potato and Asparagus Salad

Desserts/Snacks – Nutty Banana Muffins

Day 16

Breakfast – Whole Wheat Hotcakes

Lunch – Asparagus and Prosciutto in Vinegar

Dinner – Spareribs with Ginger Sauce

Desserts/Snacks – Roasted Mint Tomato Soup

Day 17

Breakfast – Cheesy Egg and Spinach on Wheat Toast

Lunch – Roasted Asparagus with Herbs and Feta Cheese

Dinner – Burrito Salad in a Jar

Desserts/Snacks – Broccoli and Turkey Muffin

Day 18

Breakfast – Nutty Banana Pancakes

Lunch – Angel Kale Puttanesca

Dinner – Zucchini, Spinach, and Tomatoes Soup

Desserts/Snacks – Baked Sweet Potato Crisps

Day 19

Breakfast – Whole Wheat Pasta and Chicken

Lunch – Creamy Tomato Broccoli

Dinner – Pumpkin Soup with Macadamia Cheese

Desserts/Snacks – Banana, Apple, and Chia Seed Parfait

Day 20

Breakfast – Scramble Tofu with Herbs

Lunch – Creamy Tomato Broccoli

Dinner – Sweet Potato and Roasted Pepper Soup

Desserts/Snacks – Avocado Quesadillas

Day 21

Breakfast – Blueberry Oatmeal

Lunch – Sweet Potato Salad in Balsamic Vinegar

Dinner – Penne Pasta with Kale

Desserts/Snacks – Pumpkin Biscuits

Day 22

Breakfast – Mixed Green Fruits Juice

Lunch – Curried Chicken

Dinner – Arugula, Corn Kernels Salad

Desserts/Snacks – Granola

Day 23

Breakfast – Broccoli Omelet

Lunch – Spanish-Inspired Scrambled Egg

Dinner – Apple Pork Stew

Desserts/Snacks – Blueberry Muffins

Day 24

Breakfast – Peaches Kiwi Shake

Lunch – Mexican-Style Salad

Dinner – Radish, Baby Greens, and Cucumber Salad

Desserts/Snacks – Egg Rolls with Lime Avocado Dip

Day 25

Breakfast – Cashew Date and Coconut Smoothie

Lunch – Curried Chicken

Dinner – Watercress, Fennel, and Apple Salad

Desserts/Snacks – Pumpkin Pie

Day 26

Breakfast – Lettuce, Avocado, and Chicken Salad

Lunch – Grilled Cauliflower

Dinner – Baked Chicken Wings in Low Fat Yogurt

Desserts/Snacks – All Fruits Salad

Day 27

Breakfast – French Toast

Lunch – Baked Marinara Turkey Meatball

Dinner – Gourmet Potato and Asparagus Salad

Desserts/Snacks – Nutty Banana Muffins

Day 28

Breakfast – Whole Wheat Hotcakes

Lunch – Asparagus and Prosciutto in Vinegar

Dinner – Spareribs with Ginger Sauce

Desserts/Snacks – Broccoli and Turkey Muffin

Day 29

Breakfast – Cheesy Egg and Spinach on Wheat Toast

Lunch – Roasted Asparagus with Herbs and Feta Cheese

Dinner – Roasted Mint Tomato Soup

Desserts/Snacks – Baked Sweet Potato Crisps

Day 30

Breakfast – Nutty Banana Pancakes

Lunch – Angel Kale Puttanesca

Dinner – Zucchini, Spinach, and Tomatoes Soup

Desserts/Snacks – Banana, Apple, and Chia Seed Parfait

CHAPTER ONE

Breakfast Recipes

French Toast

Calories 229

Total Carbohydrate 25 g

Saturated fat 2.7 g

Total Fat 11 g

Sodium 479 mg

Protein 8 g

Number of Servings: 2

Ingredients:

- 2 egg whites

- 4 slices whole wheat bread

- 1 whole egg

- ½ tsp. pure vanilla extract

- ½ cup unsweetened almond milk

- ¼ tsp. ground cinnamon

- 1/8 tsp. ground nutmeg

- Olive oil cooking spray

- ¼ tsp. brown sugar

For garnish

- pure maple syrup

- fresh fruit slices

- yogurt

Directions:

1. Beat the egg whites with the egg in a large bowl. Add the almond milk, brown sugar, cinnamon, nutmeg, and vanilla extract. Mix well.

2. Place one slice of bread into the mixture and ensure the slice is coated completely.

3. While the slice is soaking, place a non-stick skillet over medium flame and spray with some olive oil.

4. Remove the soaked slice of bread and place in the hot pan. Place the second slice in the egg mixture and allow to soak.

5. Cook the French toast for about 2 minutes per side, or until browned all over. Transfer to a platter and cook the second slice.

6.   Once both pieces of French toast are ready, serve right away. This is best served with maple syrup or yogurt and fresh fruit on top.

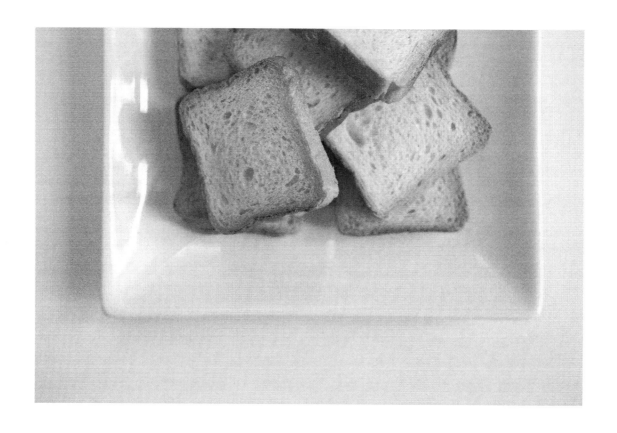

Whole Wheat Hotcakes

Calories 340

Total Carbohydrate 72 g

Saturated fat 0.4 g

Total Fat 2.5 g

Sodium 2 mg

Protein 13 g

Number of Servings: 2-4 servings

Ingredients:

- 1 cup white whole wheat flour

- 1 egg

- 6 tablespoons buttermilk powder

- ¼ cup ground flaxseed

- 1 teaspoon baking powder

- 1 teaspoon baking soda

- ½ teaspoon ground cinnamon

- 2 tablespoons canola oil

- 1 ½ cup water

- Pinch of salt

Directions:

1. In a large mixing bowl, combine the baking powder, flour, baking soda, buttermilk powder, flaxseed, and cinnamon. Beat the egg. Stir in the oil and water.

2. Add the flour mixture and whisk. Let it sit for 5 minutes.

3. Heat a griddle and coat with cooking spray. Ladle equal portions of batter onto the griddle. Cook for 2 minutes or until browned on the sides and bubbles start to form on top.

4. Flip on the other side and cook for 2 minutes.

5. Repeat steps with the other pancakes. Serve.

Cheesy Egg and Spinach on Wheat Toast

Calories 351

Total Carbohydrate 25.4 g

Saturated fat 9.8 g

Total Fat 23.6 g

Sodium 209mg

Protein 11.1g

Number of Servings: 2

Ingredients:

- 2 slices whole wheat bread

- 3 egg whites, beaten

- ¾ cup baby spinach

- 2 tomato slices

- 1 ½ tsp. brown mustard

- 2 thin slices low fat cheddar cheese

- 2 tsp. extra virgin olive oil

- Black pepper

Directions:

1. Set the oven to 400 degrees F to preheat.

2. Place a non-stick pan over medium flame and heat through. Once hot, add the olive oil and swirl to coat.

3. Add the egg whites and scramble until cooked to a desired consistency. Then, add the spinach and sprinkle in some pepper. Stir well.

4. Spread the brown mustard on one side of each slice of bread. Then, add the tomato slices on top, followed by the scrambled egg whites.

5. Add the cheese on top, then place the slices on a baking sheet. Bake for 2 minutes or until the cheese melts and the bread is lightly toasted.

6. Transfer to a serving plate and serve right away.

Nutty Banana Pancakes

Calories 227

Total Carbohydrate 30.1 g

Saturated fat 1.4 g

Total Fat 9.9 g

Sodium 287 mg

Protein 6.3 g

Number of Servings: 3

Ingredients:

- 2 egg whites

  - 1 banana, mashed

  - 1 tsp. baking powder

  - ½ cup whole wheat flour

  - 1 tsp. coconut oil, melted

  - ½ tsp. pure vanilla extract

  - Ground cinnamon, to taste

  - 1 Tbsp. walnuts, finely chopped

Directions:

⬚✍ Combine all the dry ingredients in a mixing bowl, then create a pit in the center.

⬚✍ Whisk the egg whites and milk in a separate bowl, then add the vanilla extract and mix well. Mash in the banana then stir in the coconut oil and mix well.

⬚✍ Combine the dry and wet ingredients until lumpy smooth. Do not over-mix as the pancakes will turn out tough.

⬚✍ Place a pancake griddle over medium flame and heat through. Once hot, add a bit of oil and swirl to coat.

⬚✍ Cook the pancakes until firm, about 1 minute per side, then place on a platter. Best served warm.

Whole Wheat Pasta and Chicken

Calories 176

Total Carbohydrate 27.8 g

Saturated fat 0.5 g

Total Fat 7.2 g

Sodium 130.8 mg

Protein 4.0 g

Number of Servings: 3

Ingredients:

- 4 oz. whole wheat penne pasta

- ½ cup celery, chopped

- 2 Tbsp. walnuts, chopped

- 3 oz. boneless, skinless chicken breast

- ½ cup red grapes, seedless, halved

- ¼ cup Greek yogurt, low fat, plain

- ½ Tbsp. red wine vinegar

- ¼ tsp. black pepper, freshly cracked

- Sea salt

Directions:

1. Fill a small pot with water then add a few drops of olive oil. Cover and bring to a boil over high flame.

2. Once boiling, add the whole wheat penne pasta then cook for about 8 minutes, or until al dente. Drain and set aside.

3. While the pasta is still cooking, prepare the chicken by removing any skin and excess fat. Then, slice into small cubes and set aside.

4. Boil another small pot of water over high flame and add a pinch of salt. Then, stir in the chicken cubes and cook for about 5 minutes, or until cooked through. Drain completely.

5. Place the pasta and chicken into a large bowl then add the rest of the ingredients. Turn several times to coat.

6. Cover the bowl and refrigerate for at least 1 hour before serving. Best served chilled. Store for up to 3 days in the refrigerator.

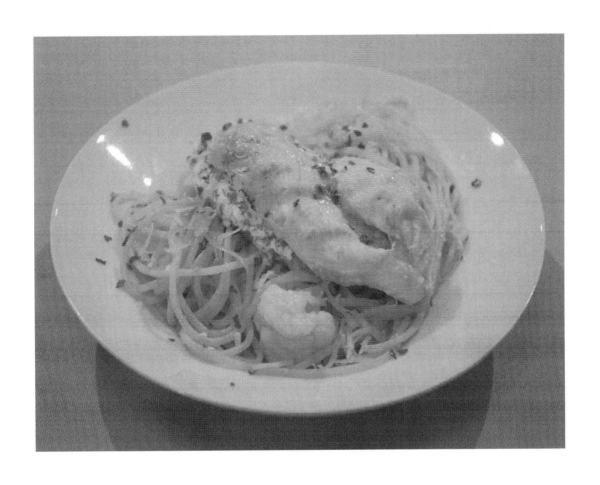

Scramble Tofu with Herbs

Calories 148

Total Carbohydrate 1.6 g

Saturated fat 3.3 g

Total Fat 11 g

Sodium 145 mg

Protein 10 g

Number of Servings: 2 servings

Ingredients:

- 1 container soft tofu

- 1 red onion, chopped

- 1 tablespoon thyme, chopped

- 1/8 teaspoon turmeric

- 1/2 cup cheddar cheese, reduced fat

- 1 tablespoon basil, chopped

- ¼ teaspoon salt

- 1/8 teaspoon pepper

- 2 tablespoons olive oil

Directions:

1. In a skillet over medium heat, heat the oil. Cook the onion for 3 minutes or until translucent. Stir in the tofu and sprinkle with, salt, pepper, and turmeric. Stir until the tofu has turned light brown.

2. Remove from heat. Add the cheese, thyme, and basil. Stir until cheese has melted.

3. Serve with wheat bread toast.

Blueberry Oatmeal

Calories 210

Total Carbohydrate 8 g

Saturated fat 0.2 g

Total Fat 7 g

Sodium 105 mg

Protein 2 g

Number of Servings: 3

Ingredients:

- 1 ½ cups fresh blueberries

- 1 ½ cups traditional rolled oats

- 2 ¼ cups almond milk, unsweetened

- 1/3 tsp. pure vanilla extract

- 3 Tbsp. pecans, chopped, toasted

Directions:

1. Pour the almond milk into a small saucepan and place over medium flame. Heat through until simmering slightly.

2. Pour in the rolled oats and stir well to combine. Continue to stir for about 3 minutes, or until the oats are tender and have absorbed most of the milk.

3. Add the blueberries into the oatmeal and stir until well-combined.

4. Divide the oatmeal among 3 bowls then sprinkle with toasted pecans on top. Best served right away.

Mixed Green Fruits Juice

Calories 201

Total Carbohydrate 4 g

Saturated fat 1.0 g

Total Fat 4 g

Sodium 102 mg

Protein 5 g

Number of servings: 5

Ingredients:

- 5 glasses of water

- 10 stalks of celery

- 5 cucumbers

- 10 green apples

- Ice

Directions:

1. Slice the apples, stalks, and cucumbers. Divide the fruits and vegetables in Ziploc bags.

2.   Refrigerate and when you need a breakfast juice, take out one plastic bag from the fridge.

3.   Place the celery, cucumbers, and apples in a blender. Add the water and ice. Serve in a glass or mason jar.

Broccoli Omelet

Calories 292

Total Carbohydrate 10.5 g

Saturated fat 5.0 g

Total Fat 11.5 g

Sodium 420 mg

Protein 25.3 g

Number of Servings: 2

Ingredients:

- 4 egg whites

- 2 garlic cloves, peeled, minced

- 2 whole eggs

- ¾ cup broccoli, chopped

- ½ cup feta cheese, low fat

- ¼ tsp. chilli pepper flakes

- 3 Tbsp. extra virgin olive oil

- black pepper, freshly cracked

Directions:

1. Whisk the egg whites and eggs in a large bowl until smooth.

2. Place a large non-stick pan over medium flame and heat through. Once hot, add 1 ½ tablespoons of the olive oil in the pan.

3. Once the pan is hot, stir in the broccoli and sauté until tender. Then, stir in the garlic and chilli pepper flakes. Mix well then season with black pepper.

4. Continue to sauté until the broccoli is crisp tender. Transfer to a bowl and set aside.

5. Wipe the non-stick pan over medium flame and heat through over medium flame again. Add the remaining olive oil and swirl to coat.

6. Add the egg mixture and tilt several times until the egg is evenly cooked.

7. Flip over the omelette and then add the broccoli mixture and feta cheese on half of the omelette.

8. Fold over the omelette and cover the pan. Turn off the heat and allow the cheese to melt for about two minutes.

9. Transfer the omelette to a serving dish and slice in half. Best served right away.

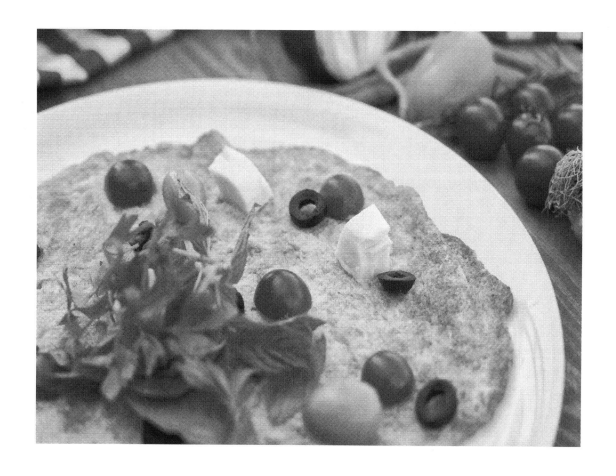

Spanish-Inspired Scrambled Egg

Calories 468

Total Carbohydrate 25 g

Saturated fat 12 g

Total Fat 29 g

Sodium 1 mg

Protein 28 g

Number of Servings: 2

Ingredients:

- 1 egg

- 2 egg whites

- 1 green bell pepper, diced

- 1 tomato, chopped

- 1 green onion, chopped

- 2 Tbsp. unsweetened soy milk

- ground black pepper

- Hot sauce

- Olive oil

Directions:

1. Lightly coat a skillet with cooking spray and place over medium flame.

2. Once hot, add the tomato, bell pepper, and green onions. Saute until crisp tender. Transfer to a bowl and set aside.

3. Beat the egg with the egg whites in a bowl then add the soy milk and whisk well. Season with black pepper to taste.

4. Pour the egg mixture into the hot pan and scramble until slightly firm but still moist. Stir the vegetables back into the pan with the eggs.

5. Transfer the egg scramble to a serving dish and serve right away.

Peaches Kiwi Shake

Calories 116.8

Total Carbohydrate 32.4 g

Saturated fat 0.4 g

Total Fat 0.9 g

Sodium 49.1mg

Protein 4.1 g

Number of Servings: 2

Ingredients:

- 2 cups peaches sliced, frozen

- 2 cups peeled kiwifruit

- 2 cups frozen strawberries

- 2 Tbsp. pure maple syrup

- 4 cups ice cubes

- 1 ½ cups chilled coconut water

Directions:

1.   Combine all the ingredients in a high power blender and cover securely.

2.   Blend on low until the ingredients a shredded, then increase to medium speed and blend until smooth.

3.   Pour into two tall glasses and consume right away.

Cashew Date and Coconut Smoothie

Calories 187

Total Carbohydrate 31.8 g

Saturated fat 0.6 g

Total Fat 2.7 g

Sodium 61.2 mg

Protein 11.1 g

Number of Servings: 2

Ingredients:

- 12 cashew nuts

- 1 frozen banana

- 4 cups ice cubes

- 1 cup unsweetened almond milk

- 1 cup chilled coconut water

- 2 Tbsp. raw cashew butter

- 2 Tbsp. chopped pitted Medjool dates

- 2 tsp. chopped lemongrass

- 2 tsp. pure vanilla extract

Directions:

1. Combine all the ingredients in a high power blender and cover securely.

2. Blend on low until the ingredients a shredded, then increase to medium speed and blend until smooth.

3. Pour into two tall glasses and consume right away.

Lettuce, Avocado, and Chicken Salad

Calories 450.5

Total Carbohydrate 10.0 g

Saturated fat 10.7 g

Total Fat 24.6 g

Sodium 423 mg

Protein 46.8 g

Number of Servings: 2

Ingredients:

- 1 head romaine lettuce, chopped

- 1 tomato, diced

- ½ small avocado

- 4 oz. cooked chicken breast, shredded

- 1 hard-boiled egg, chopped

- 1 small cucumber, seeded and sliced

- 1 cooked turkey bacon, crumbled

For the Dressing

- 2 Tbsp. water

- 2 Tbsp. crumbled blue cheese

- 1 ½ Tbsp. white wine vinegar

- ½ Tbsp. minced shallot

- ½ tsp. Dijon mustard

- ¼ tsp. freshly ground black pepper

Directions:

1. First make the dressing by combining the water, vinegar, mustard, shallot, and black pepper in a bowl. Whisk well to combine.

2. Add the blue cheese to the dressing and stir gently to combine. Set aside.

3. Put the lettuce in a mixing bowl and drizzle in half the dressing. Toss well to coat.

4. Divide the lettuce into two servings then top with the chicken, tomato, egg, and cucumber.

5.   Remove the stone from the avocado and scoop out the flesh. Then, slice into small cubes and place on the salad. Sprinkle the turkey bacon on top and add the remaining dressing. Best served right away.

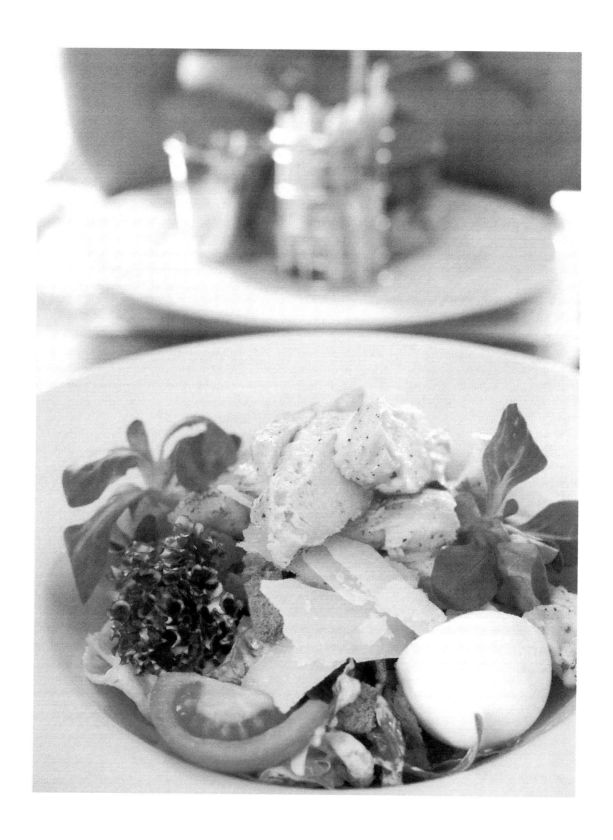

CHAPTER TWO

Lunch Recipes

Baked Marinara Turkey Meatball

Calories 249

Total Carbohydrate 10.8 g

Saturated fat 2.9 g

Total Fat 10.8 g

Sodium 208.1 mg

Protein 24.6 g

Number of Servings: 3

Ingredients:

- 1 egg

- ¾ lb. lean ground turkey

- 3 Tbsp. feta cheese, low fat

- 1 garlic clove, diced

- 1 red onion, diced

- 1 red bell pepper, stemmed, seeded, diced

- 12 oz. organic marinara sauce, low sodium

- 3 Tbsp. whole wheat bread crumbs

- 1/3 tsp chili pepper flakes

- 1/3 tsp. dried Italian herbs

- 1/8 tsp. ground cumin

- 2 Tbsp. fresh flat leaf parsley, chopped

- Freshly ground black pepper

- 3 Tbsp. extra virgin olive oil

Directions:

1. Set the oven to 375 degrees F to preheat.

2. Mix together the ground turkey, onion, garlic, bell pepper, parsley, chili pepper flakes, cumin, and Italian herbs in a large mixing bowl. Add the egg and black pepper and mix well with clean hands.

3. Divide the turkey mixture into small, 1 inch meatballs and arrange on a platter. Set aside.

4. Place a large non-stick skillet over medium high flame and heat through. Once hot, add the olive oil and swirl to coat.

5. Cook the turkey meatballs in the skillet until browned all over, then transfer to a baking dish. Arrange in a single layer.

6. Pour the marinara sauce over the turkey meatballs then cover the dish with aluminium foil.

7. Bake for 20 minutes. Then, uncover and top with feta cheese. Bake for an additional 3 minutes.

8. Remove from the oven and then let stand for 5 minutes. Best served warm.

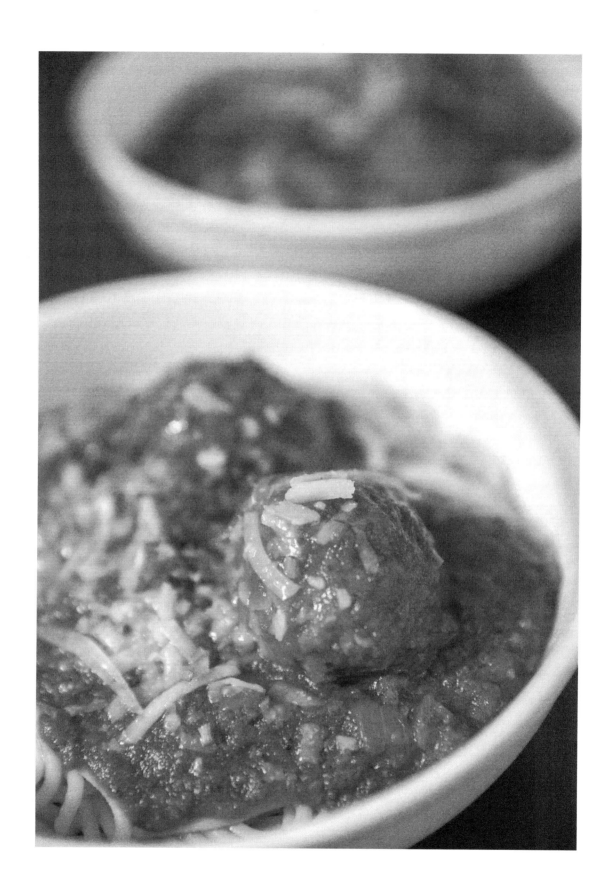

Asparagus and Prosciutto in Vinegar

Calories 56.2

Total Carbohydrate 3.7 g

Saturated fat 1.2 g

Total Fat 3.7 g

Sodium 267 mg

Protein 3.9 g

Number of Servings: 3

Ingredients:

- 3 bunches asparagus, trimmed

- 6 prosciutto

- 250 grams cherry tomato, finely chopped

- 1 tablespoon white wine vinegar

- 2 anchovy fillets, chopped finely

- 1/3 cup pine nuts, toasted

- Pinch of salt

- Pinch of pepper, to taste

- Pinch of sugar

- 2 tablespoons olive oil

Directions:

1. Preheat oven to 400°F. Then, use non-stick baking paper to line baking tray. Place prosciuttos on the tray. Bake until crisp (around 5 minutes). Set aside to cool slightly (around for 5 minutes), and then use fingers to break prosciuttos into large pieces.

2. For the dressing, whisk tomato, anchovy, vinegar, olive oil and sugar together in a small bowl. Add salt and pepper to taste.

3. Preheat chargrill or barbecue grill on high settings. Brush asparagus with olive oil. Add salt and pepper to taste. Cook asparagus on grill, occasionally turning (usually after about two minutes), or until tender crisp and bright green.

4. To serve, divide asparagus among plates. Drizzle with the dressing and then top with crispy prosciuttos and pine nuts.

Roasted Asparagus with Herbs and Feta Cheese

Calories 55.4

Total Carbohydrate 3.2 g

Saturated fat 0.6 g

Total Fat 4.7 g

Sodium 98.5 mg

Protein 1.4 g

Number of Servings: 4

Ingredients:

- 2 pounds asparagus

- 4 garlic cloves, minced

- 1/4 teaspoon red pepper flakes

- ½ teaspoon dried oregano

- 1/4 cup olive oil

- 1 teaspoon lemon zest

- 1 lemon

- 2 tablespoons fresh Italian parsley, chopped

- Pinch of salt

- Pinch of ground black pepper

- 4 oz crumbled feta cheese

Directions:

1. Preheat oven to about 400 degrees F.

2. Heat oil in a small pan on low heat settings, and then add garlic, red pepper flakes, lemon zest and oregano. Remove from heat when the olive oil becomes fragrant and the garlic turns golden in color. Allow to cool.

3. Bend asparagus spears gently until they snap at the natural point. Throw away the ends.

4. Drizzle the olive, garlic and lemon zest mixture over the asparagus. Toss to coat pieces evenly.

5. On a baking sheet with a side age, place spears in one layer. Add kosher salt and black pepper to taste. Sprinkle feta cheese on top.

6. Roast asparagus for about 12 minutes or until desired tenderness is achieves

7. Top with parsley. Squeeze lemon over the roasted asparagus, but make sure to catch the seeds. Serve.

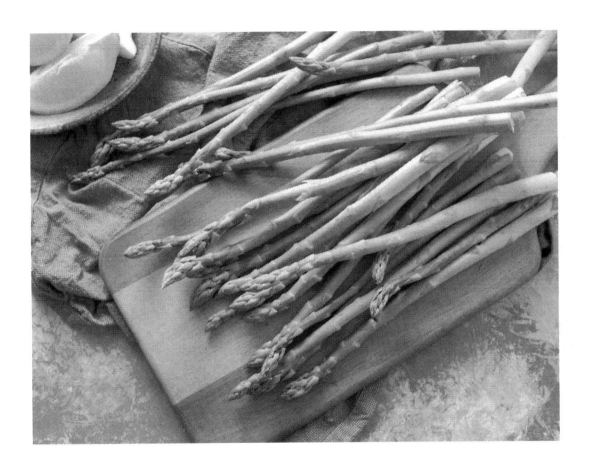

Angel Kale Puttanesca

Calories 580

Total Carbohydrate 93 g

Saturated fat 2.3 g

Total Fat 15 g

Sodium 290 mg

Protein 1.6 g

Number of Servings: 4

Ingredients:

- 16 oz angel hair pasta

- 2 garlic clove, minced

- ½ onion, sliced

- 1 can black olives, drained

- 2 tablespoons olive oil

- 1 tablespoon capers, drained

- ½ cup Parmesan cheese, grated

- 1 teaspoon red pepper flakes

- 1 can anchovy fillets, drained

- 2 cups kale, chopped

- 1 cup diced tomatoes, do not drain

Directions:

1. Prepare the pasta by cooking it in a pot of lightly salted water. Place the pasta in the water when it starts to boil. It should be done in about ten minutes.

2. In a separate pan, cook the garlic, onions and red pepper flakes in a skillet containing olive oil on medium heat. When the ingredients turn brown, throw in the anchovy and tomatoes. Allow to simmer. Reduce the flame to medium and add the kale. Cook for an additional ten minutes.

3. Drain the pasta when done and throw it into the pan with the olive oil. Toss the pasta in the oil and serve with a sprinkle of Parmesan cheese.

Creamy Tomato Broccoli

Calories 65.2

Total Carbohydrate 12.7 g

Saturated fat 0.4 g

Total Fat 1.1 g

Sodium 297 mg

Protein 2.4 g

Serving size: 4

Ingredients:

- 4 cups dry broccoli slaw

- 1 teaspoon garlic, chopped

- ¼ cup water

- Dash of crushed red pepper

- 1 cup creamy tomato soup, low fat

- 3 tablespoons parmesan cheese, grated

- 1 dash onion powder

- Pinch of salt

- Pinch of black pepper

Directions:

1. In a skillet medium-high heat, prepare a nonstick pan.

2. Add the broccoli slaw and pour ¼ cup water. Allow the broccoli to cook for 7 minutes whilst stirring occasionally. All the water should have evaporated.

3. Add the red pepper, black pepper, creamy tomato sauce, 2 tablespoons parmesan cheese, onion powder, garlic, and salt. Cook for 5 minutes whilst stirring.

4. Sprinkle with the remaining parmesan cheese before serving.

Sweet Potato Salad in Balsamic Vinegar

Calories 138.2

Total Carbohydrate 18.2 g

Saturated fat 4.1 g

Total Fat 6.9 g

Sodium 234 mg

Protein 2.2 g

Number of Servings: 3

Ingredients:

- 1 lb. sweet potato, peeled and sliced into cubes

- 1 celery stalk, diced

- ½ Tbsp. shallots, minced

- 1 tsp. fresh chives, chopped

- 1 ½ Tbsp. balsamic vinegar

- ½ Tbsp. apple cider vinegar

- 1 tsp. fresh parsley, chopped

- ½ tsp. Dijon mustard

- ¼ tsp. raw honey

- ¼ tsp. freshly ground black pepper

- 2 Tbsp. olive oil

Directions:

1. Arrange the potatoes in a pot and add just enough water to cover by about 2 inches. Cover the pot and place over high flame then bring to a boil.

2. Once boiling, reduce to medium low flame and simmer until the potatoes are fork tender.

3. Meanwhile, prepare the dressing by combining the honey, mustard, balsamic and cider vinegars in a salad bowl and whisk well to combine. Add the olive oil and whisk again to combine.

4. Add the celery, chives, parsley, shallots, and pepper in the vinaigrette. Toss well to coat.

5. Once the potatoes are ready, drain them and place in a salad bowl.

6. Pour the dressing with the herbs and chives on top of the potatoes, then serve.

Curried Chicken

Calories 73

Total Carbohydrate 7 g

Saturated fat 0 g

Total Fat 3 g

Sodium 56 mg

Protein 4 g

Serving size: 2-4 servings

Ingredients:

- 2 chicken breast, sliced into strips

- ½ eggplant, chopped

- 3 garlic cloves, minced

- 2 cups chicken broth

- 2 green bell peppers, chopped

- 1 zucchini, sliced into thick strips

- 2 tsp dried oregano leaves

- 1/3 cup raisins

- 1 tsp curry powder

- 2 cups tomatoes, chopped

- 1 potato, cut into wedges

- ½ tsp turmeric

- ¼ cup black olives, sliced

- 1 Tbsp. vegetable oil

Directions:

1. Rinse eggplant in cold water in a colander.

2. Cook peppers, garlic, onion and vegetable oil in an oven over medium heat for around 3 minutes or until tender. Stir frequently.

3. Add eggplant, potato, zucchini, tomato, raisins, oregano, curry powder, turmeric and olives. Bring to a boil and then reduce heat.

4. Simmer and cover for about25 minutes or just until vegetables become tender.

5. Add chicken strips and then cook for around 4 minutes before serving.

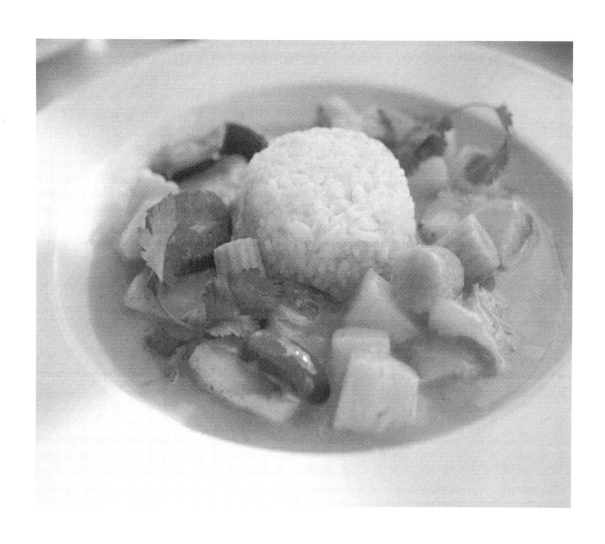

Grilled Cauliflower

Calories 271

Total Carbohydrate 9 g

Saturated fat 15.6 g

Total Fat 25.2 g

Sodium 143 mg

Protein 5.8 g

Serving size: 2 servings

Ingredients:

- 1 pound fresh cauliflower, cut into slabs

- 3 tablespoons light soy sauce

- 1 lemon juice

- 1 tablespoon sesame oil

- Vegetable oil, for grilling

Directions:

1. Marinate cauliflower using the lemon juice and soy sauce. Set aside for 5 to 10 minutes.

2. Place a skillet over medium heat. Drizzle the skillet with oil. Arrange the marinated cauliflower in the skillet. Grill on each side for 5 to 10 minutes depending on the size of the slabs.

3. After all the slabs are grilled, sprinkle the sesame oil over them and toss until all the slabs are evenly coated with oil.

Heirloom Tomatoes and Ruby Beets Salad

Calories 82.5

Total Carbohydrate 13.1 g

Saturated fat 0.5 g

Total Fat 3.6 g

Sodium 25.4 mg

Protein 1.1 g

Number of Servings: 3

Ingredients:

- 3 beets, trimmed

- ¾ cup green heirloom tomatoes, sliced

- 4 cups mixed greens

- 3 Tbsp. balsamic vinegar

- 3 Tbsp. walnuts, toasted, chopped

- 3 Tbsp. goat cheese, crumbled

- Freshly ground black pepper, to taste

Directions:

1. Arrange the beets in a small pot and fill the pot with about a cup of water. Cover and place over medium high flame then cook for 15 minutes, or until tender.

2. Once the beets are cooked, drain and slice into quarters. Place in a large mixing bowl and set aside.

3. Slice the heirloom tomatoes and add to the bowl of beets, followed by the walnuts and goat cheese.

4. Add the balsamic vinegar and toss well to coat. Then, season with black pepper and toss again to combine.

5. Divide the salad into individual servings. Best served right away.

Kale and Mango Salad

Calories 84

Total Carbohydrate 3.9 g

Saturated fat 0.9 g

Total Fat 7.3 g

Sodium 58 mg

Protein 1.5 g

Serving size: 2 servings

Ingredients

- 1 Handful of kale

- 1 mango, diced

- 1 lemon, freshly juiced

- pumpkin seeds, toasted

- 2 tablespoons honey

- Pinch of salt

- Pinch of ground black pepper

- Extra virgin olive oil

Directions:

1. Mix some olive oil, kosher salt, lemon juice and kale in a large bowl. Tenderize the kale leaves by massaging in the oil and the other ingredients. That will take about 5 minutes.

2. In a separate bowl, combine honey, pepper and some more lemon juice. That will serve as the dressing for the salad.

3. Combine the kale and the dressing by pouring the honey mixture over the leaves. Garnish the salad with the mango fragments and the pumpkin seeds. Be sure to mix before serving.

Wheat Tortillas with Peppers and Mushrooms

Calories 304

Total Carbohydrate 39.8 g

Saturated fat 2.8 g

Total Fat 14.9 g

Sodium 413 mg

Protein 8.0 g

Serving size: 2-4 servings

Ingredients:

- 5 whole wheat flour tortillas

- 3 tablespoons olive oil

- 1 onion, thinly sliced

- 1 red bell pepper, thinly sliced

- 1 green bell pepper, thinly sliced

- 3 Portobello mushrooms caps, thinly sliced

- 1 teaspoon chili powder

- 1/3 teaspoon cumin

- 4 tablespoons salsa

- 2 tablespoons vegan sour cream

Directions:

1. In a skillet over medium heat, pour the olive oil.

2. Sauté the onion, bell peppers, and mushrooms until tender. Sprinkle chili powder and cumin. Mix well. Remove from the pan and set aside.

3. To serve, layer the mushrooms and peppers on warmed tortillas. Toast for 3 minutes. Add vegan sour cream on top. Serve.

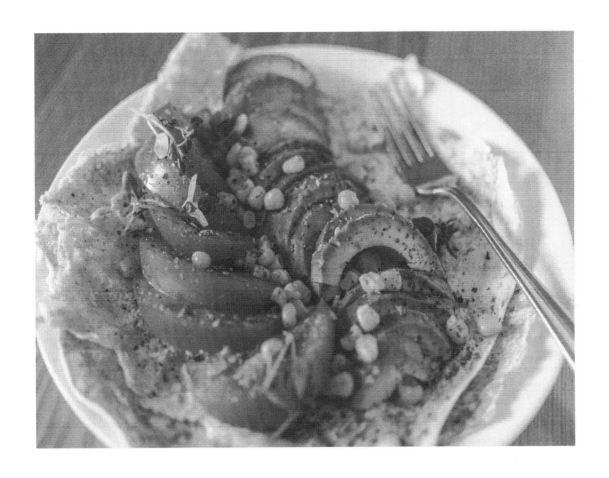

Artichoke and Spinach Soup

Calories 47

Total Carbohydrate 11 g

Saturated fat 0 g

Total Fat 0.2 g

Sodium 94 mg

Protein 3.3 g

Serving size: 2-4 servings

Ingredients:

- 2 tablespoon non-dairy butter

- ½ cup non-dairy cream

- 1 small garlic clove, minced

- ½ onion, minced

- 1 celery stalk, diced

- 2 cups vegetable broth

- 1 can artichoke hearts, drained, quartered

- 2 handfuls fresh spinach leaves

- ¼ teaspoon xanthan gum

- 1 tablespoon lemon juice, freshly squeezed

- Pinch of sea salt

- Pinch of ground black pepper

Directions:

1. Put the artichoke hearts into a food processor and add ¼ cup of the vegetable broth and the xanthan or guar. Blend until pureed.

2. Place a non-stick skillet over medium flame and heat through. Once hot, reduce to medium flame and add the butter, onion and celery. Sauté until onion becomes tender.

3. Add the garlic and sauté until fragrant. Spoon in the artichoke puree, then add the remaining broth. Increase to medium high flame and let simmer.

4. Stir in the cream and lemon juice, then season to taste with salt and pepper. Serve right away or chilled.

CHAPTER THREE

Dinner Recipes

Gourmet Potato and Asparagus Salad

Calories 120

Total Carbohydrate 10 g

Total Fat 0.7 g

Sodium 89 mg

Protein 3.2 g

Saturated fat 0 g

Serving size: 4 servings

Ingredients:

- 2 cups potatoes, sliced diagonally

- 2 bunches asparagus, ends trimmed, halved diagonally

- 1/4 cup buttermilk

- 1 can green peppercorns, drained, rinsed, coarsely chopped

- 1/3 cup mayonnaise

- 1 tablespoon vinegar

- 1 tablespoon fresh dill, chopped finely

- an 80-gram packet of baby rocket leaves

- Pinch of salt

- Pinch of ground black pepper

Directions:

1. In a large saucepan, place potatoes and then pour a good amount of cold water until covered. Place pan over high heat and then bring to a boil. Cover pan and then cook until tender (usually takes around 8 minutes). Rinse potatoes through cold running water, and then thoroughly drain.

2. While cooking the potatoes, place salted water in a medium saucepan. Bring to a boil and then place for asparagus pieces. Cook for 2-3 minutes or until tender crisp and bright green. Run cold water over spears and then thoroughly drain.

3. In a bowl, place buttermilk, mayonnaise, vinegar, dill and peppercorn. Whisk with a fork until thoroughly mixed. Taste and add salt and pepper as desired.

4. In a serving bowl (large), place the asparagus, potato, and rocket leaves and then gently toss to combine ingredients. Lightly pour mayonnaise mixture. Serve while freshly made.

Spareribs with Ginger Sauce

Calories 254

Total Carbohydrate 12 g

Total Fat 2.8 g

Sodium 120 mg

Protein 6.5 g

Saturated fat 2.0 g

Serving size: 4 servings

Ingredients:

- ½ teaspoon Chinese five-spice powder

- ½ teaspoon ground coriander

- 1 teaspoon brown sugar

- ½ teaspoon salt

- ¼ teaspoon pepper

- 2 lbs spareribs

- ½ cup apricot jam

- 2 tablespoons rice vinegar

- ¼ cup ginger, minced

- ¼ cup soy sauce, low sodium

- ¼ teaspoon red pepper, crushed

Directions:

1.   Preheat the oven to 35o degrees F.

2.   For the rubs, combine five-spice powder, coriander, brown sugar, salt, and pepper in a bowl. Rub onto the ribs. Roast for 1 hour.

3.   Meanwhile, preheat the grill over high heat.

4.   For the sauce, combine apricot jam, rice vinegar, ginger, soy sauce, and red pepper in a saucepan. Bring mixture into a boil. Transfer to a bowl.

5.   From the oven, put spareribs on the grill rack, baste with apricot jam, and grill for 7 minutes. Cut the rack into individual ribs. Serve with sauce.

Roasted Mint Tomato Soup

Calories 86

Total Carbohydrate 6.5 g

Total Fat 0.1 g

Sodium 35 mg

Protein 2.1 g

Saturated fat 0.2 g

Number of Servings: 6

Ingredients:

- 9 cups vegetable broth, low sodium

- 4 ½ lb. plum tomatoes, halved

- 2 small yellow onions, chopped

- 2 cups fresh mint, chopped

- 1/3 cup lemon juice, freshly squeezed

- 4 Tbsp. olive oil

- 2 tsp. freshly ground black pepper

Directions:

1. Set the oven to 400 degrees F to preheat.

2. Combine the tomatoes, garlic, and onion in a baking sheet. Add the olive oil and toss to coat. Sprinkle in the black pepper and toss again to combine.

3. Spread the tomatoes in a single layer, cut side facing up, then roast for 45 minutes in the oven or until extra tender.

4. Place the roasted tomatoes in a food processor or blender and blend until smooth. Then, pour into a stock pot and stir in the broth.

5. Place the pot over high flame and bring to a boil. Once boiling, reduce to low flame and stir in the lemon juice. Mix well.

6. Add the chopped fresh mint and stir well to combine. Ladle into soup bowls and serve right away. Soup may be stored in individual containers in the freezer for up to 3 months.

Burrito Salad in a Jar

Calories 150

Total Carbohydrate 6.5 g

Total Fat 13 g

Sodium 35 mg

Protein 3 g

Saturated fat 0.2 g

Number of Servings: 5

Ingredients:

- 2 chicken

- 2 cups quinoa cooked

- 2 cups bacon, crumbled

- 1 sweet potatoes, cubed

- 1 tablespoon coconut oil

- ½ cup of cilantro, chopped

- ¾ cup of cheese, shredded

- 5 tablespoons plain Greek yogurt

- 3 cups of lettuce, chopped

- Pinch of salt

- Pinch of pepper

Directions:

1. Season the chicken with salt and pepper. In large pan, heat one tablespoon of coconut oil over medium heat. Add the chicken and cook for four minutes each side. Remove the chicken from the pan and let it cool on a chopping board.

2. Add one tablespoon of Greek yogurt at the bottom of the mason jar. Add the sweet potato cubes. Add three tablespoons of quinoa and one tablespoon of cilantro.

3. Add two tablespoons of cheese. Add bacon. Top with lettuce. Serve and enjoy.

Zucchini, Spinach, and Tomatoes Soup

Calories 283

Total Carbohydrate 50.5 g

Saturated fat 1.3 g

Total Fat 7.2 g

Sodium 287 mg

Protein 6.6 g

Number of Servings: 3

Ingredients:

- 1 zucchini, diced

- 5 oz frozen spinach, chopped

- 1 can diced tomatoes, juices reserved

- 1 onion, chopped

- 1 ½ quarts vegetable broth

- 1 tablespoon dried basil

- 1 green bell pepper, diced

- 1 cup firm tofu, cubed

- 2 garlic cloves, minced

- 1 carrot, diced

- 1 celery stalk, diced

- 1 tablespoon dried oregano

- 1 teaspoon ground black pepper

- 4 oz non-dairy cheese, shredded

- 2 tablespoon chipotle peppers in adobo sauce, vegan, chopped

- 1 ripe avocado

- 2 tablespoons olive oil

Directions:

1. Place a soup pot over medium flame and heat through. Once hot, add the oil and swirl to coat.

2. Sauté the onion, carrot, zucchini, and celery until tender. Add the bell pepper and garlic and sauté until fragrant.

3. Add the basil, oregano, and black pepper, then sauté until fragrant. Pour in the broth, and tomato with juices.

4. Reduce to low flame and simmer for 20 minutes.

5. Add the tofu and frozen spinach, then boil for an additional 5 minutes.

6. To serve, divide the cheese and chopped chipotle peppers among five bowls. Pour the soup over the cheese and pepper mixture.

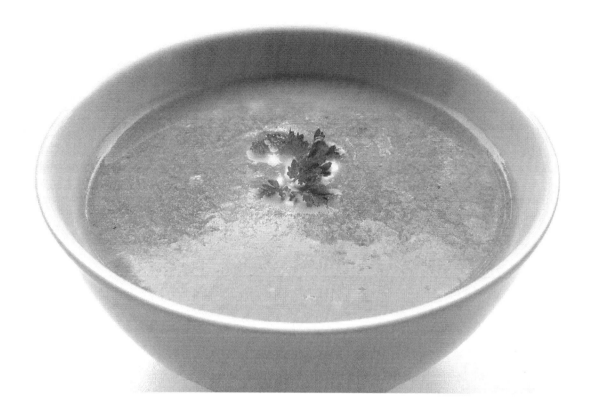

Pumpkin Soup with Macadamia Cheese

Calories 71

Total Carbohydrate 11.03 g

Saturated fat 1.5 g

Total Fat 2.5 g

Sodium 586 mg

Protein 2.5 g

Number of Servings: 4

Ingredients:

- 2 cans pumpkin puree, unsweetened

- 1 white onion, minced

- 1 garlic cloves, minced

- 4 cups   vegetable stock

- 1 tablespoon olive oil

- Pinch of salt

- Pinch of white pepper

For garnish

- 1 tablespoon shelled pumpkin seeds

- ¼ cup   macadamia nut cheese with sun-dried tomatoes

- ¼ cup   fresh chives, minced

Directions:

1. Pour oil into Dutch oven set over medium heat. When oil is hot enough, add in and sauté onion and garlic until limp and aromatic.

2. Except for garnishes, add in remaining ingredients. Stir. Bring soup to a boil. Secure lid. Turn down heat. Simmer for 20 minutes. Turn off heat.

3. Cool slightly before processing into a blender until smooth. Taste; adjust seasoning, if needed.

4. Cool slightly before ladling into bowls. Add equal portions of garnishes on top.

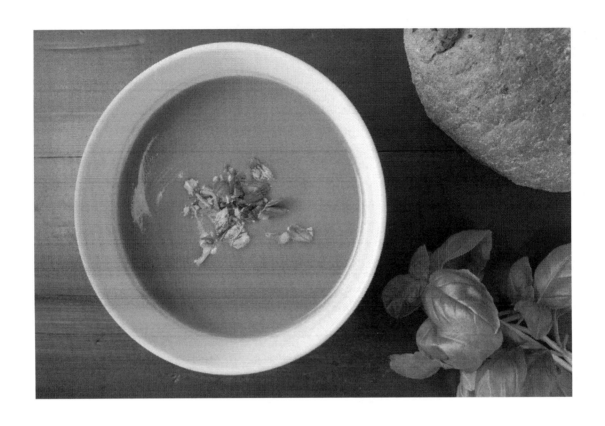

Sweet Potato and Roasted Pepper Soup

Calories 104.4

Total Carbohydrate 21.9 g

Saturated fat 0.5 g

Total Fat 1.0 g

Sodium 286 mg

Protein 2.3 g

Number of servings: 2

Ingredients:

- 2 tablespoons olive oil

- 2 red peppers

- 1 sweet potato, cubed

- 2 garlic cloves, minced

- 2 cups vegetable broth

- ¼ cup sweet basil, julienned

- ½ cup onion, chopped

- ½ cup carrots, chopped

- ½ cup celery, chopped

- ½ cup coconut milk

- Pinch of sea salt

- Pinch of ground pepper

Directions:

1. Place the oven into the 375 degrees F.

2. Combine the onions and sweet potatoes on a baking sheet. Add the red peppers beside the mixture. Drizzle some of the olive oil over everything and toss well to coat.

3. Roast for 20 minutes, or until sweet potatoes are golden and peppers are tender and skins are wilted.

4. Chop the roasted red peppers and set aside.

5. Place a pot over medium high flame and heat through. Once hot, add the olive oil and swirl to coat.

6. Place the carrot, celery, and garlic into the pot and sauté until carrot and celery are tender. Add the chopped roasted red peppers and sweet potato-onion mixture. Mix well.

7.   Pour in the vegetable broth and coconut milk. Increase to high flame and bring to a boil.

8.   Once boiling, reduce to a simmer. Simmer, uncovered, for 10 minutes.

9.   Season to taste with salt and pepper, then turn off the heat and allow to cool slightly.

10. If desired, blend the soup using an immersion blender until the soup has reached a desired level of smoothness. Reheat over medium flame.

11. Add the basil and stir to combine. Serve right away.

Penne Pasta with Kale

Calories 283

Total Carbohydrate 50.5 g

Saturated fat 1.3 g

Total Fat 7.2 g

Sodium 287 mg

Protein 6.6 g

Number of Servings: 3

Ingredients:

- 2 tablespoons olive oil

- 3 cups penne pasta, uncooked

- ½ teaspoon salt

- 1 sliced medium onion

- 8 thinly sliced garlic cloves

- 6 cups kale

Directions:

1. Cook the onions in a skillet with oil until they turn brown. Be sure to stir the onions as they cook to prolong the cooking time. After fifteen minutes of cooking, add the garlic and cook for another 2 minutes.

2. In a separate saucepan, prepare the Penne pasta as indicated by the packaging instructions. Use lightly salted water to cook the pasta.

3. In another separate area, boil enough water to submerge the kale. Cover the lid and allow the kale to cook for about fifteen minutes or until the kale becomes soft. Be sure to drain the kale when done.

4. Take the cooked Penne, drained and place on a serving platter. Pour the onion and oil mixture unto the Penne. Finally, throw in the softened Kale.

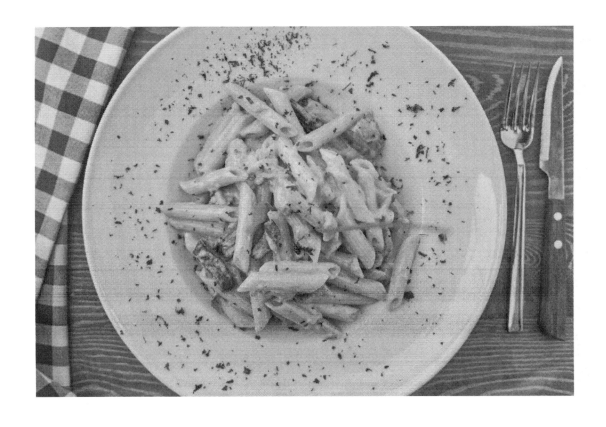

Arugula, Corn Kernels Salad

Calories 191

Total Carbohydrate 3 g

Saturated fat 1 g

Total Fat 1.0 g

Sodium 206 mg

Protein 6 g

Number of serving: 2-4 servings

Ingredients:

- ½ cup   fresh arugula leaves, torn

- ½ cup   canned whole corn kernels, drained

- ½ cup canned white beans, drained

- 1 head   endive, torn

- 1 stalk leek, minced

For the dressing

- 1 teaspoon extra virgin olive oil

- 3 teaspoons apple cider vinegar

- 1 Dijon mustard

- Pinch of kosher salt

- Pinch of white pepper

Directions:

1.   In a bottle with tight fitting lid, combine olive oil, apple cider vinegar, mustard, salt, and pepper. Seal and shake well bottle until well blended.

2.   In a salad bowl, put arugula leaves, corn kernels, white beans, endive, and leek. Drizzle the dressing.

3.   Place equal portions into salad bowls. Serve.

Apple Pork Stew

Calories 242

Total Carbohydrate 32 g

Saturated fat 1.9 g

Total Fat 5.4 g

Sodium 123 mg

Protein 16.5 g

Number of Servings: 3

Ingredients:

- 2 green apple, chunked

- 1 onion, diced

- 1 lb. boneless pork shoulder, sliced into thin strips

- ½ lb. new potatoes, scrubbed clean

- 2 slices turkey bacon

- ½ cup green cabbage, shredded

- ¾ cup apple juice

- 1 ½ Tbsp. Dijon mustard

- ¾ Tbsp. white wine vinegar

- ¾ Tbsp. fresh thyme leaves

- 1/3 tsp. freshly ground black pepper

- 1 ½ Tbsp. canola oil

Directions:

1. Place a heavy duty stock pot over medium high flame and heat through. Once hot, add the onions and sauté until golden brown.

2. Add the pork and sauté until the pork is browned all over. Then, transfer everything to a large bowl and set aside.

3. In the same pot, add the potatoes, apple, cabbage, apple juice, broth, mustard, and pepper. Stir well then increase to high flame and bring to a boil.

4. Once boiling, reduce to medium low flame and simmer. Then, return the pork and onions and add the vinegar and bacon. Simmer for 15 minutes.

5. Ladle into soup bowls and top with thyme. Best served right away.

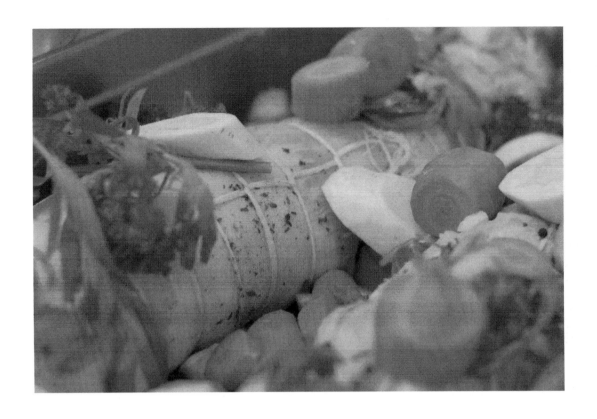

Mexican-Style Salad

Calories 316.6

Total Carbohydrate 50.7 g

Saturated fat 1.4 g

Total Fat 7.4 g

Sodium 649.3 mg

Protein 14 g

Number of Servings: 3

Ingredients:

- 3 Roma tomatoes, chopped

- ¾ cup cucumber, sliced

- 3 cups romaine lettuce, chopped

- 1 white onion, sliced thinly

- 2 ½ Tbsp. lime juice, freshly squeezed

- 2 Tbsp. extra virgin olive oil

- Pinch of sea salt

- Pinch of ground black pepper, to taste

Directions:

1. Place the lettuce into a large salad bowl, then add the cucumber, onion, and tomatoes.

2. Drizzle in the olive oil and the lime juice, then toss everything to combine.

3. Season to taste with salt and pepper, then toss again. Divide into individual servings and serve right away.

Radish, Baby Greens, and Cucumber Salad

Calories 48

Total Carbohydrate 9 g

Saturated fat 0 g

Total Fat 0 g

Sodium 106 mg

Protein 3 g

Number of Servings: 2

Ingredients:

- 6 oz. mixed baby greens

- 2 radishes, sliced thinly

- 1 red bell pepper, stemmed, cored, seeded and diced

- 1 cucumber, halved and sliced thinly

For the Vinaigrette

- 1 small red onion, peeled and minced

- 1 Tbsp. rice vinegar

- 1 Tbsp. canola oil

- ¾ Tbsp. freshly grated ginger

- ½ Tbsp. organic low sodium ketchup

- ½ Tbsp. organic low sodium soy sauce

- ½ tsp. sesame oil

Directions:

1. First make the dressing by combining the vinegar, canola oil, ginger, onion, ketchup, sesame oil, and soy sauce. Mix well and set aside.

2. Combine the baby greens, cucumber, radishes, and bell pepper in a salad bowl and toss to combine.

3. Drizzle in dressing over the salad and toss again to coat. Serve.

Watercress, Fennel, and Apple Salad

Calories 138.7

Total Carbohydrate 9 g

Saturated fat 0.1 g

Total Fat 2.3 g

Sodium 320 mg

Protein 4 g

Number of servings: 2 servings

Ingredients:

- ½ cup watercress, shredded

- 1 apple, diced

- 1 bulb fennel, julienned

- ¼ cup   pine nuts, freshly toasted

Dressing

- 1 teaspoon Dijon mustard

- ¼ teaspoon basil, dried

- 1 teaspoon extra virgin olive oil

- 3 teaspoon apple cider vinegar

- Pinch of salt

- Pinch of pepper

Directions:

1. In a bottle with tight fitting lid, combine olive oil, apple cider vinegar, Dijon mustard, basil, salt, and pepper. Seal and shake bottle until well blended.

2. In a salad bowl, put together apple, bulb fennel, watercress, and pine nuts. Drizzle the dressing.

3. Place equal portions into salad bowls. Serve.

Baked Chicken Wings in Low Fat Yogurt

Calories 128

Total Carbohydrate 1.2 g

Saturated fat 2.2 g

Total Fat 11 g

Sodium 50 mg

Protein 16 g

Number of servings: 3-4

Ingredients:

- 2 lbs chicken wings

- 5 sprigs fresh thyme

- 5 cloves garlic, crushed

- 1 cup Greek yogurt, low-fat

- ½ cup blue cheese, crumbled

- Pinch of salt

- Pinch of ground pepper

- ¾ cup hot sauce

Directions:

1. Preheat the oven to 375 F. Grease a baking pan.

2. Meanwhile, in a bowl, out chicken wings.

3. Prepare a skillet over low heat. Saute garlic and thyme for 4 minutes. Allow to simmer for 3 minutes. Pour hot sauce. Stir well.

4. Add the mixture over the chicken and toss until well-coated.

5. In another bowl, combine Greek yogurt and blue cheese. Mix well and refrigerate. Bake the chicken for 30 minutes.

6. Remove from the oven. Allow the chicken to cool for few minutes Baste chicken wings juices. Serve with dip.

Grilled Chicken with Kale Salad

Calories 226

Total Carbohydrate 15 g

Saturated fat 3.9 g

Total Fat 15 g

Sodium 235mg

Protein 23 g

Number of servings: 2

Ingredients

- 2 chicken breasts, boneless, skinless

- ½ pound red-skinned potatoes, cut into smaller pieces

- 3 garlic cloves, thinly sliced

- ½ cherry tomatoes, halved

- 1 tablespoon lemon juice, freshly squeezed

- 1 handful of kale

- 4 cups mixed salad greens

- 2 tablespoons extra virgin olive oil

- Pinch of salt

- Pinch of ground pepper

Directions:

1. Pour some of the olive oil in a baking sheet. Place the potato pieces in the sheet and toss. Make sure that all the pieces are covered in the olive oil. Roast the potatoes in an oven pre-heated to 218C for five minutes.

2. In a separate bowl, combine the salt, pepper kale, half a teaspoon of olive oil and garlic. Toss the kale in the mixture until the leaves are fully coated.

3. Throw the kale into the same baking sheet with the potatoes and place it back in the oven to bake for about 20 minutes. The kale should be crispy by that time.

4. In a separate pan, pour or brush some olive oil and heat over a medium flame. When hot, cook the chicken. Make sure to cut the chicken horizontally to make 4 smaller sections and then coat each section in olive oil, salt and pepper.

5. Remove the potatoes and the kale from the oven and continue to toss them in the remaining amount of olive oil in another bowl. Serve the chicken with the kale salad on the side.

Tofu Platter

Calories 76

Total Carbohydrate 1.9 g

Saturated fat 0.7 g

Total Fat 4.8 g

Sodium 7 mg

Protein 8 g

Number of servings: 2

Ingredients:

- 6 oz tofu, cut into pieces

- 1 tomato, chopped

- ¼ cup capers

- 1 Tbsp. Greek seasoning

- 1 jar kalamata olives, pitted

- 1 Tbsp. lemon juice

- 1 onion, chopped

- ¼ cup olive oil

- Pinch of salt

- Pinch of pepper

Directions:

1. Pre-heat oven to 350 degrees.

2. Put the tofu in an aluminum foil sheet and season with Greek seasoning. Combine capers, olives, tomato, lemon juice, olive oil, salt and pepper in a bowl then spoon the tomato mixture over the halibut.

3. Seal edges of the foil sheet carefully so that you'll be able to make a large packet. Place the said packet on a baking sheet.

4. Bake for around 30 to 45 minutes or until fish flakes are easily crumbled by a fork. Serve and enjoy.

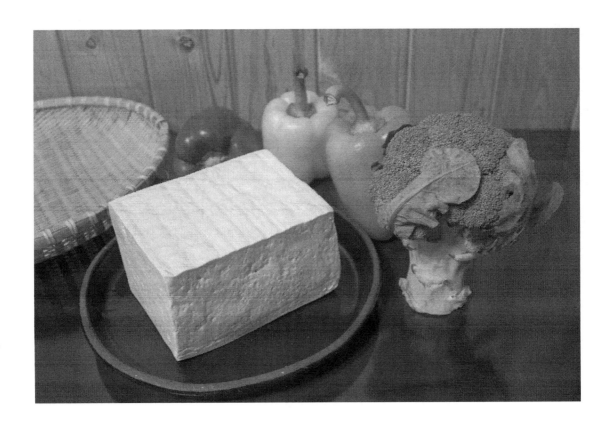

Beans Pasta Soup

Calories 249

Total Carbohydrate 49.1 g

Saturated fat 1.2 g

Total Fat 2.1 g

Sodium 309 mg

Protein 14.4 g

Number of servings: 2-4 servings

Ingredients

- 2 cups pasta, cooked

- 1 can cannellini beans, drained

- 2 cups spinach, chopped coarsely

- 2 bay leaves

- 1/2 tsp. dried sage

- 4 tbsps. Romano cheese, grated

- 1 can diced tomatoes

- 1 cup onion, chopped

- 1 celery stalk, chopped

- 1 zucchini, chopped

- 1 tsp. dried thyme

- 3 cups vegetable stock, reduced-fat

- 1/2 tsp. dried sage

- Pinch of salt

- Pinch of ground black pepper

Directions:

1. Combine tomatoes, celery, carrots, beans, sage, thyme, bay leaves and broth in a slow cooker.

2. Season with half-teaspoon each of salt and pepper.

3. Cook in low setting for maximum of 8 hours or maximum of 4 hours on high.

4. Add vegetables and pasta 30 minutes before the stock ingredients are cooked.

5. Cover and continue cooking or 30 minutes.

6. Remove and discard bay leaves.

7. Season again with salt and pepper according to desired taste.

8. Ladle soup into individual bowls and top each with parmesan cheese.

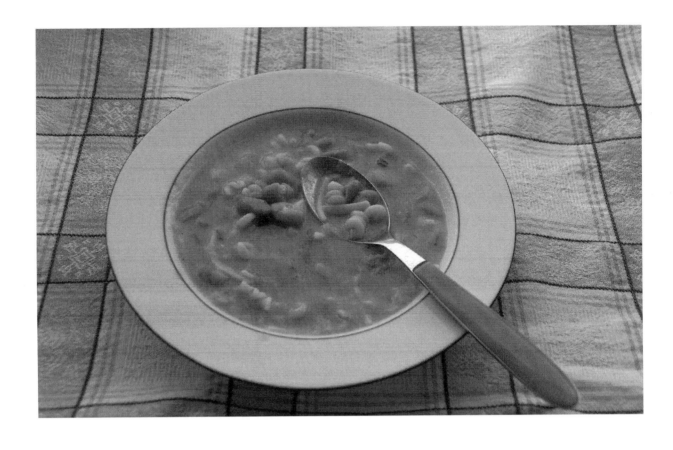

CHAPTER FOUR

Dessert and Snacks Recipes

Nutty Banana Muffins

Calories 286

Total Carbohydrate 36.4 g

Saturated fat 6.5 g

Total Fat 14.6 g

Sodium 143 mg

Protein 4.4 g

Number of servings: 4

Ingredients:

- 2 eggs

- 1 1/2 tsps. baking soda

- 2 cups all-purpose flour

- 4 bananas, overripe

- ½ cup brown sugar

- 1/2 cup pecans, chopped

- 3/4 cup butter, unsalted, melted

- 1 tsp. vanilla extract

- 1/2 tsp. salt

Directions:

1. Preheat oven to 375 degrees Fahrenheit.

2. Grease muffin cups on two muffin pans.

3. Combine flour, salt and baking soda in a large bowl. Mix well by using a pastry blender or fork. Set aside.

4. Mash two bananas using a fork in a bowl.

5. Mix the remaining two bananas and sugar using a handheld or counter top electric mixer for 3 minutes.

6. Add vanilla, eggs and melted butter to the banana-sugar mixture. Beat well. Scrape sides of the bowl to place the ingredients near to the mixing blade.

7. Add dry ingredients then blend. Pour mashed bananas and pecans to the mixture. Fold using a rubber spatula.

8. Scoop the batter into muffin cups. Fill each cup halfway Nudge the pan on the countertop to eliminate air bubbles.

9. Cook for 20 minutes or until cake tester or a barbecue stick comes out clean when the muffin is pierced.

10.   Take the pan out to cool and serve at room temperature or warm.

Broccoli and Turkey Muffin

Calories 338

Total Carbohydrate 2 g

Saturated fat 5.4 g

Total Fat 21 g

Sodium 366 mg

Protein 21 g

Number of servings: 2

Ingredients:

For the muffins

- 8 eggs

- 2 cups broccoli, finely chopped

- ¼ cup sun-dried tomatoes in oil, chopped finely

- ½ teaspoon onion powder

- 1 cup cheddar cheese, shredded

- ¼ teaspoon dried oregano

- 1 teaspoon dried basil

- ½ teaspoon salt

- 1 tablespoon chives

For the sausage

- ½ lb turkey meat

- 1 tablespoon olive oil

- 1 teaspoon fennel seeds

- 1 garlic clove, minced

- 1 teaspoon dried parsley

- ½ onion, finely chopped

- 1 teaspoon dried oregano, crumbled

- 1 teaspoon dried basil

- ½ teaspoon salt

- ½ teaspoon ground black pepper

Directions:

1. Preheat the oven to 350 F. Grease a muffin pan.

2. Meanwhile, cook the garlic and onion in a pan over medium heat for 3 minutes. Remove and set aside.

3. In a large bowl, combine the onion mixture with the beef. Then, add in the oregano, fennel seeds, basil, parsley, black pepper, and sea salt. Mix using your hands to form meat patties.

4. Preheat the pan over medium heat and cook the patties for 7 minutes. Cook until the meat is no longer pink in color. Set aside and let cool. Chop into bite-size pieces.

5. Meanwhile, in another mixing bowl, combine the broccoli, cheese, oregano tomatoes, basil, onion powder, salt, and cooked meat.

6. In a separate bowl, whisk the eggs. Pour into the broccoli with meat mixture and combine. Divide into even portions and pour into the muffin cups. Top each cup with chives.

7. Place into the oven and bake for 30 minutes. Put in the cooling rack and let cool completely.

Baked Sweet Potato Crisps

Calories 162.5

Total Carbohydrate 36.7 g

Saturated fat 0.1 g

Total Fat 0.9 g

Sodium 15.1 mg

Protein 2.6 g

Number of Servings: 4

Ingredients:

- 2 sweet potatoes, peeled, thinly sliced

- Olive oil

- 2 tsp. fresh rosemary, minced

Directions:

1. Set the oven to 400 degrees F to preheat.

2. Lightly coat 4 baking sheets with olive oil cooking spray then arrange the sliced sweet potato on top.

3. Spray the slices of sweet potato with olive oil cooking spray once again. Sprinkle the rosemary on top.

4. Bake the sweet potato crisps for 15 minutes or until crisps. Place on the cooling rack and allow to cool to touch.

5. Serve right away or store in an airtight container at room temperature for up to 2 days.

Banana, Apple, and Chia Seed Parfait

Calories 259

Total Carbohydrate 48.6 g

Saturated fat 0.4 g

Total Fat 5.2 g

Sodium 2.1 mg

Protein 5.9 g

Number of servings: 2-4

Ingredients:

For the Parfait base

- 1 overripe banana, mashed

- 2 tablespoons chia seeds

- ½ teaspoons cinnamon powder

- 1¼ cups almond milk, chilled

- ⅛ teaspoon nutmeg powder

For the Apple jam

- 2 apples, diced

- 2 tablespoons chia seeds

- ¾ cup   organic apple juice, unsweetened

- ⅛ teaspoon nutmeg powder

- ¾ teaspoons cinnamon powder

- Pinch of sea salt

- 1 tablespoon cashew nuts, chopped, for garnish

Directions:

1. Mix parfait base ingredients in a bowl. Chill in fridge until ready to assemble.

2. Place apple jam ingredients in a thick-bottomed saucepan set over medium heat; boil. Reduce heat; place lid on.

3. Simmer for 25 minutes, stirring once in a while. Turn off heat. Using a potato masher, mash half of jam. Set aside to cool completely to room temperature.

4. To assemble: alternately spoon 2 tablespoons of both parfait base and apple jam into 2 tall parfait glasses until filled almost to the top.

5. Garnish with cashew nuts if using; serve.

Avocado Quesadillas

Calories 297

Total Carbohydrate 32.5 g

Saturated fat 1.8 g

Total Fat 18.1 g

Sodium 205 mg

Protein 6.7 g

Number of servings: 2

Ingredients:

- 4 whole wheat flour tortillas

- 1 avocado, ripe, chopped

- 1 1/2 cups cheese, shredded

- 1/4 cup sour cream

- 2 ripe tomatoes, chopped

- 1 red onion, medium-sized, chopped

- 3 tablespoons fresh coriander, chopped

- 1/4 teaspoon Tabasco sauce

- Pinch of salt

- Pinch of pepper

- 1/2 teaspoon vegetable oil

- 2 teaspoons lemon juice, freshly squeezed

Directions:

1. In a small to medium mixing bowl, combine the avocado, Tabasco, tomatoes, onion, and lemon juice. Mix well. Add salt and pepper to taste.

2. In a small bowl, mix the coriander, sour cream, and then add a pinch of salt and pepper.

3. Place tortillas on a baking sheet and brush the ops with oil. Broil around 2 to 4 inches from heat until they become pale golden in color. Sprinkle evenly with shredded cheese and then broil again until cheese melts.

4. Spread the first mixture (avocado) evenly over two tortillas and then use remaining tortillas (cheese side facing down) to top those. This would make 2 quesadillas. Transfer them to a cutting board and ten slice into 4 wedges.

5. Use a dollop of the second mixture (the one with sour cream) to top each wedge. Serve warm.

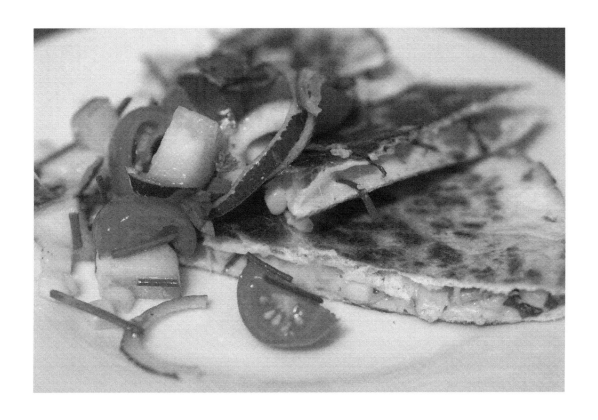

Pumpkin Biscuits

Calories 259

Total Carbohydrate 48.6 g

Saturated fat 0.4 g

Total Fat 5.2 g

Sodium 2.1 mg

Protein 5.9 g

Number of servings: 2-4

Ingredients:

- 1 1/4 teaspoons pumpkin pie spice

- 2 cups all-purpose flour

- 2 1/2 teaspoons baking powder

- 3 tablespoons of honey

- 1/3 cup buttermilk, fat-free

- 5 tablespoons butter, chilled, cut into small pieces

- 3/4 cup of canned pumpkin

- 1/2 teaspoon salt

Directions:

1. Preheat oven to a temperature of 400°F.

2. Weigh flour or lightly spoon into a dry measuring cup and then level using a knife.

3. In a large bowl, mix flour, salt, pumpkin pie spice, and baking powder. Use a pastry blender (2 knives if you do not have one) to cut in butter until the mixture looks like coarse meal and then chill mixture for about 10 minutes.

4. Mix honey and buttermilk by using a whisk to stir until thoroughly blended. Then, add canned pumpkin. Add this mixture to the chilled flour mixture. Stir mixture until it's moist.

5. Prepare a lightly floured surface. Turn dough out into that and then lightly knead 4 times to ensure that biscuits would be tender. Roll dough into a half-inch-thick rectangle measuring 9 x 5 inches.

6. Dust the top of the dough with flour and then fold crosswise into thirds (like you would with a piece of paper to make it fit inside an envelope). Then, reroll the dough into a rectangle that's the same size as before. Dust the top with flour again. Fold the dough

into thirds, crosswise this time and then gently pat or roll until its ¾ inch thick.

7. Use a 1 3/4-inch biscuit cutter to cut dough, making14 dough rounds. Line a baking sheet with parchment paper. Place dough rounds about an inch apart on a baking sheet lined and then bake at a temperature of 400°F until golden brown, or around 14 minutes. Remove biscuits from the pan and then place on wire racks for 2 minutes to cool. These biscuits are best served warm.

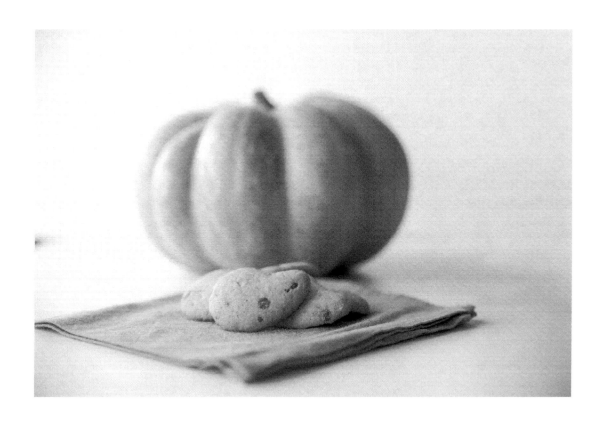

Granola

Calories 471

Total Carbohydrate 64 g

Saturated fat 2.4 g

Total Fat 20 g

Sodium 294 mg

Protein 10 g

Number of servings: 2-4

Ingredients:

Base

- 1 cup almond flour, finely milled

- ¼ cup raw organic honey

- ½ cup almond flour, coarsely milled

- 2 tsp. cinnamon powder

- ½ tsp. pure maple syrup, optional

- 1 tsp. sea salt

- ½ cup coconut oil

- 2 tsp. vanilla extract

Flavorings

- 1 Tbsp. chia seeds

- Pinch sesame seeds

- 1 dried date, deseeded, minced

- 1 Tbsp. sunflower seeds, roasted and shelled

- ⅛ cup walnuts, chopped

- ⅛ cup pecans, chopped

Directions:

1. Preheat the oven to 275°F. Line a baking dish with parchment paper. Overhangs on the side are required for easier lifting of the baked granola.

2. For the flavorings, using the Instant Pot Pressure Cooker, press the "saute" button. Cook dried dates, sunflower seeds, chia seeds, sesame seeds, walnuts, and pecans. Toast until aromatic and light brown in color. Remove from the instant pot and set aside.

3. To make the granola, using a large mixing bowl, put together almond flour, cinnamon powder, honey, vanilla extract, salt, and coconut oil. Mix well. Press into the baking dish. Bake for 15 minutes or until a toothpick inserted comes out clean.

4. Remove from the oven. Cool the granola before placing in cake rack. Slice into bite-sized squares. Serve.

Blueberry Muffins

Calories 57

Total Carbohydrate 14 g

Saturated fat 0 g

Total Fat 0.3 g

Sodium 1 mg

Protein 0.7 g

Number of servings: 4

Ingredients

- 2 1/2 cups blueberries

- 2 eggs

- 2 cups all-purpose flour

- 1/2 cup milk

- 2 tsps. baking powder

- 1 tsp. vanilla

- 1 cup sugar

- 1/2 cup butter, low fat, set at room temperature

- 1/4 tsp. salt

For garnish

- 1/4 tsp. ground nutmeg

- 1 tbsp. granulated sugar

Directions:

1. Preheat oven to 375 degrees Fahrenheit.

2. Mix granulated sugar and nutmeg in a small bowl. Mix well. Set aside.

3. Grease a muffin pan with 18 regular-sized cups or 12 large-sized cups

4. Cream butter or margarine using a wooden spoon or a rubber spatula in a bowl.

5. Stri in sugar to the butter and continue creaming until fluffy.

6. Tip in one egg at a time. Mix each time you place an egg. Add salt, baking powder and vanilla.

7. Add half of milk and flour into the batter. Fold and add the remaining flour and milk. Continue folding until well blended.

8. Stir in blueberries. Fold to blend well. Scoop the batter into muffin cups.

9. Top each muffin with a sprinkle of sugar-nutmeg topping. Bake for 20 minutes until muffin is fluffy, moist and golden brown.

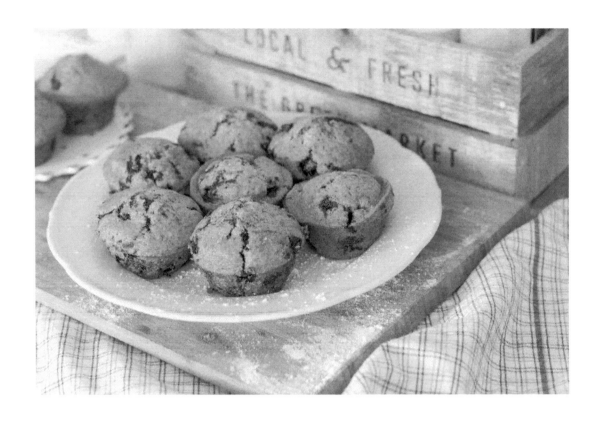

Egg Rolls with Lime Avocado Dip

Calories 196

Total Carbohydrate 29 g

Saturated fat 1 g

Total Fat 4.5 g

Sodium 378 mg

Protein 10 g

Number of servings: 2

Ingredients:

- 20 egg roll wrappers

- 2/3 cup corn

- 2 1/2 cups chicken, cooked, shredded

- 2/3 cup canned black beans, drained

- 1 1/2 cups Mexican cheese blend , shredded

- 1/4 cup fresh cilantro, minced

- 1/4 teaspoon of cayenne pepper

- 1 teaspoon of lime peel, grated

- Oil

- 1 teaspoon of ground cumin

- 5 green onions, chopped

- 1 teaspoon of salt

For the dip

- 1 tablespoon fresh cilantro, minced

- 1 ripe avocado, mashed

- 1 cup ranch dressing

- 1 teaspoon lime peel, grated

Directions:

1. Combine the first ten ingredients in a large bowl. Mix well. Cover wrappers with a damp paper towel.

2. To place filling for every egg roll wrapper, place 1/4 cup of the mixture right in the center. Keep the remaining wrappers covered while you make one egg roll after another.

3. To wrap, fold the bottom corner of the wrapper over the filling. Then, fold the sides toward the middle, over the filling. Use water to moisten remaining side. To seal, roll tightly. Repeat process until you're done with the rest of the mixture

4. Heat oil on a deep-fat fryer or electric skillet at 375 degrees F.

5. Fry only a few egg rolls at a time until they are golden brown for – each side should take about 2 minutes. Drain on paper towels.

6. For the dip, combine the four ingredients for the dip. Mix thoroughly. Serve with egg rolls.

Pumpkin Pie

Calories 243

Total Carbohydrate 35 g

Saturated fat 2 g

Total Fat 10 g

Sodium 239 mg

Protein 3.9 g

Number of servings: 4-6

Ingredients:

- 2 eggs

- 1 can pumpkin

- 1/8 teaspoon ground cloves

- 1 teaspoon ground cinnamon

- 1/3 cup shortening

- ½ cup sugar

- ½ teaspoon salt

- 1 can evaporated milk

- ½ teaspoon ground ginger

- 1 cup all-purpose flour

- 1 tablespoon sugar

- 3 tablespoons cold water

Directions:

1. Combine the flour and salt in a bowl then add the shortening. Use two knives to pull the ingredients to turn them into small peas.

2. Drizzle some cold water on the peas to make sure that the flour becomes moist and that none of the flour sticks to the bowls and stays in the pastry.

3. Shape the resulting material into a ball. This can be done on a surface covered in flour. This dough should then be covered in a plastic wrap and left in the refrigerator for about an hour.

4. Before baking, use a rolling pin to flatter the dough into a wide enough circle to cover a pie plate. This will serve as the base of the pie. Be sure to trim leftover dough hanging from the edge of the pie plate.

5. In a separate bowl, throw in all the remaining ingredients along with the beaten eggs to create the pie filling. That includes the sugar, salt, evaporated milk, pumpkin, cinnamon and ginger. Beat these ingredients together until the individual ingredients are indistinguishable.

6. In an oven pre-heated to 425F, place the pie plate. Reduce the oven to 350F while baking. Allow it to bake for forty five minutes. Let the pie cool for about half an hour. Store in refrigerator for about 4 hours. For best results, leave overnight.

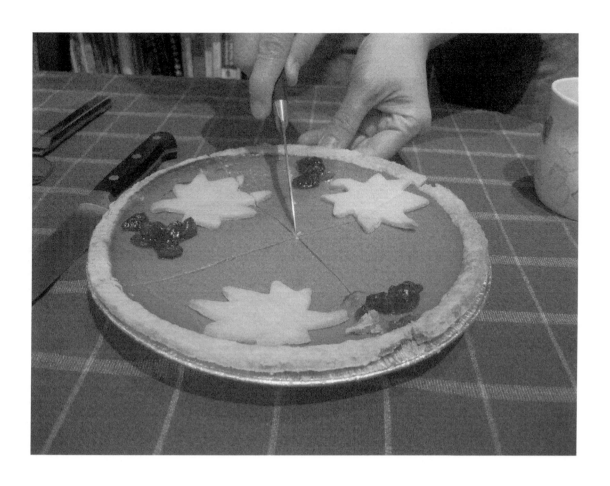

All Fruits Salad

Calories 152

Total Carbohydrate 15 g

Saturated fat 1.6 g

Total Fat 10 g

Sodium 203 mg

Protein 1 g

Number of servings: 2

Ingredients:

- 1 banana, sliced into thick disks

- 1 mango, diced

- 2 tablespoon lime juice, freshly juiced

- ¼ cup   ripe jackfruit, deseeded, diced

- ¼ cup   canned pineapple tidbits, drained

- 1 teaspoon cashew nuts, freshly toasted

- 1 tablespoon raw sugar cane

Directions:

1. In a bowl, mix lime juice and sugar cane. Shake well until the sugar dissolves.

2. In another bowl, put the mango, banana, pineapple tidbits, jackfruit, and cashew nuts. Drizzle the dressing. Toss well to combine.

3. Place equal portions into bowls. Serve.

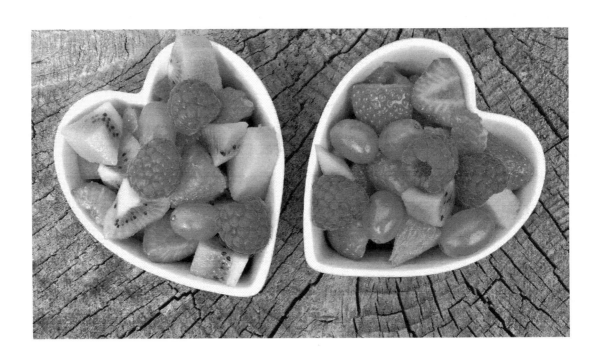

Avocado with Ginger Smoothie

Calories 258

Total Carbohydrate 26.8 g

Saturated fat 2.1 g

Total Fat 14.4 g

Sodium 42.7 mg

Protein 9.6 g

Number of servings: 2

Ingredients:

- 1 pitted avocado, halved

- 1 teaspoon soy sauce

For garnish

- cilantro

- pickled ginger

- wasabi

Directions:

1. Place spoon between avocado skin and meat to loosen.

2. Pour half a teaspoon of soy sauce over each avocado half.

3. Use spoon to scoop meat out.

4. Add ginger, cilantro or wasabi to taste.

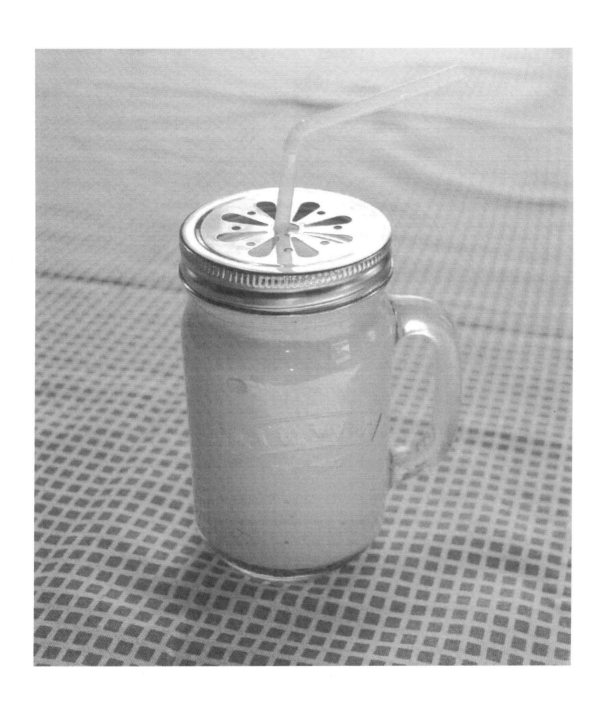

BONUS CONTENT

MEAL PREP CHAPTER 2

On Mindful Eating and Curbing Hunger

Switching to a healthier lifestyle, especially after you've been used to doing things a particular way for so long will take some adjustment. There will be challenges and you might find yourself falling behind at certain points—understand that this is totally fine. What matters is that you get back on track, exert a bit more effort, and make some necessary changes that will support the kind of life you want to have.

When it comes to eating healthier, it's more than just selecting the right food and doing portion control. Your overall mental approach matters just as much and being mindful about how you do things can really help make things easier. With that said, here are a few Do's and Don'ts to keep in mind.

The Do's

4. Do start with your shopping list.

Always take your time and make sure you feel focused when writing your list. Mindfulness is key when it comes to creating the right grocery list that will benefit your goals. Think about how you've been feeling lately—what does your body require at the moment? With that in mind, start putting together your choices and edit it as you go.

5. Do savor your meals.

Here's the thing, most people actually rush through their meals because of various reasons. Some may not have a lot of time to spare, whilst there are those who want to use that time for something else "more important". However, it is important to relish your food; take the time to enjoy its flavor, its aroma, and chew properly. Eating mindfully also makes you feel sated for a longer period of time.

6. Do the "mouth full, hands empty" mantra.

This means that you should set your cutlery down in between mouthfuls of food. Quite similar to the previous tip, this is meant to help slow your eating and enable you to better appreciate your food. Not only that, doing this can actually help increase the response of your gut peptides. You'll feel full for longer and keep you from overeating.

7. Always wait a minute or two before going back for seconds.

This allows the food you just ate to settle down and give you enough time to think if you really want more. Most people have a tendency to immediately go for seconds right after eating, especially if the food is something they really like. However, this often leads to them feeling too full and bloated. So, take your time after finishing your plate. Have some water or a sip of tea, then decide if you really need to refill your plate.

8. Do keep your bigger serving bowls of food off the table and out of sight.

This is to serve the previous step's purpose. If you cannot immediately see or reach the food, you won't be able to refill your plate quickly. It also keeps you from craving more just because you keep seeing food. As you may or may not know, just the mere visual of delicious food can make us overeat. If we can see it and smell even while eating, we're bound to grab more servings.

The Don'ts

9. Don't eat while you're distracted by something.

A lot of us fall into the trap of multi-tasking; in this case, eating whilst doing something else. Maybe you do it while you're watching TV, while you're working, or while you're moving from one place to the next. Sure, it feels good to be accomplishing a lot of things at the same time, but did you know that this can be detrimental to your fitness goals? By doing this, you're likelier to overeat or end up snacking again later. This is because your brain isn't fully processing the fact that you're eating.

So next time, give yourself an hour or 30 minutes to eat your meals.

10. Don't drink too much alcohol before you begin eating.

Aside from its calorie content, research has shown that people who drink more before eating are actually more prone to cheating on their diets. Alcohol is also known to stimulate are appetites, making it harder for us to say no to food we cannot have.

11.   Don't eat when you're feeling stressed.

A lot of us have a tendency to "eat our feelings" as a means of relieving stress or any emotional distress we may be experiencing. Whilst this does seem to work, it can also cause us to overeat and feel guilty later on. Instead of turning to food during stressful moments, try mindfulness meditation instead. This will help turn our attention away from what we're craving (usually very indulgent food items) and is also a healthier alternative to stress eating.

12.   Don't forego your diet just because you're eating out.

As we've already established, there are ways of still following your diet even when you're out with friends. Remember, people also tend to eat more when they're in social settings or surrounded by friends. Don't stress yourself out when the menu for an event or a restaurant does not fit into your WW freestyle diet. Where you might not be able to be pickier of what you eat, you can always opt for portion sizes.

Eating mindfully is one thing, but the real challenge often happens when you're trying to beat hunger. It can make just about anyone restless and even cranky—everyone's familiar with this. Here are a few do's and don'ts to keep in mind when it comes to curbing your hunger:

The Do's

13.	Do your best to always get enough sleep.

Not getting enough sleep actually affects the balance of your hormones related to the appetite. Research shows that people who have had less than 5 hours of sleep experienced an increase in the ghrelin levels in their body. This is the hormone which actually triggers appetite and decreases leptin levels. Leptin is the hormone that signals our brain when we've had enough food.

14.	Do a bit of cardio after eating.

Doing this has a positive effect on our satiety hormones, helping promote a longer feeling of satiety. Research also proves that doing moderate-intensity exercises can curb feelings of hunger. It is also an effective form of distraction, keeping you from unintentionally eating or snacking.

When you start feeling the need to snack, try going for a walk instead. After you get back from it, you're bound to feel less inclined to grab a bag of chips or snack on your favorite treats. Note that the brain actually enjoys when we form new habits so do try and focus on making healthier ones, instead of trying to break your current bad habits. You'll eventually replace them when the good habits stick.

15. Do have a hearty breakfast.

Breakfast is important—essential to our day. Having a hearty one provides our body with the ample fuel it needs to give you a head start on the day. People who begin their day with a protein-rich breakfast are less likely to begin craving snacks halfway through their morning. It also keeps you from overeating when lunchtime comes around, effectively preventing body fat gain and enabling you to manage your hunger better.

The Don'ts

16. Don't eat too many fatty foods.

Having too much dietary fat in your daily meals can actually trigger ghrelin, the hunger hormone. Basically, the fattier the food you eat is, the greater your appetite for it would become. Just think back to all the times you've eaten food like French fries, pizzas, steaks, and so on—it's usually really hard to stop, right? This is why.

Another thing to pay attention to is your low-fat food's total energy content. These type of food is likely to contain great amounts of sugar to compensate for any flavor that's lost due to the low-fat content.

17. Don't deprive yourself of your favorite foods.

It's totally okay to enjoy the foods you love, but make sure you do so moderately. Doing so actually helps you deal with cravings better and makes you feel less guilty about having them as well. Banning a food only serves to increase your craving for it so don't be afraid to have your favorites whenever you really feel like them.

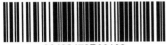

36493479R00109

Made in the USA
San Bernardino, CA
22 May 2019